# **Hormone Reset Diet**

Proven Step by Step Guide to Cure Your Hormones, Balance your health, and Secrets for Weight Loss up to 5LBS In 1 Week

# Table Of Contents

Hormone Reset Diet

Introduction

Chapter 1: Hormonal Imbalance: The Root Cause of Weight Loss Problems

Chapter 2: Basics of Hormone Reset Diet

Chapter 3: Metabolic hormones in the body and their role in Weight Loss

Chapter 4: How to Repair Hormones and Lose weight in the Process through Hormone Reset Diet

Chapter 5: The Hormone Diet: Indepth Review

Chapter 6: Sample Hormone Reset Diet Recipes

# Introduction

I want to thank you and congratulate you for downloading the book, *"Hormone Reset Diet"*.

This book contains proven steps and strategies on how to repair your hormone imbalances, improve your general health, and lose weight of up to 5 pounds in just a week.

Hormones play a vital role in our everyday lives. They are the reason why we feel energized. They cause positive and negative mood swings especially in women. Interestingly, hormones also affect the way we look at ourselves. Balanced hormones level in the body keeps us lean, strong and sexy.

Forget about age problems. Let us not use aging as an excuse for feeling unattractive or for having not-so-great sex with our partner. Hormones affect all these. If you want to feel young or if you want to have better sex, you need to have balanced hormones. How do we achieve that?

Diet is the key. Everything that we eat affects the hormone levels in the body. When we feel that we are gaining weight, our first tendency is to reduce the amount of food that we eat. This drastic change in the eating pattern creates stress in the body which sends our metabolic hormones flying in all directions. Cortisol, a stress hormone will cause you to crave comfort foods resulting to unwanted belly fat even in people who are otherwise skinny.

This book will help you achieve that. Here's what you will find inside:

- Information about the different important hormones in the body
- Step by step guide on how to balance hormone levels in the body
- Roles that hormones play in the improvement of one's growth and development
- Tips on how to lose weight in as little as 1 week through the hormone reset diet
- Details about the hormone reset diet and how effective it is
- Sample recipes for the hormone reset diet

Thanks again for downloading this book, I hope you enjoy it!

## Chapter 1: Hormonal Imbalance: The Root Cause of Weight Loss Problems

Have you ever wondered why none of the dietary programs you have tried really worked well for you? Do you still gain weight despite all your hard work in keeping yourself fit? Do you easily feel stressed out with simple things? If you answered "yes" to all these questions, then you have failed to address the real root cause of the problem—hormonal imbalance.

Here are some questions that you need to ask yourself first to help determine if you have imbalanced hormones or not:

- Do you usually feel a strong urge to eat sweets or carbs at 3pm?
- Do you find it difficult to get yourself out of bed in the morning?
- Do you easily get irritated even by simple things?
- Do have mood swings?
- Do you experience pre-menstrual syndrome every month?
- Do you have trouble getting a good night's sleep?
- Is your skin dull and dry?
- Do you have a belly fat that you can't seem to get rid of no matter what you do?
- Do you always feel bloated after every meal?

If your answer is "yes" to all of these questions, then your hormone levels are not balanced. Fortunately, this book was written specifically for you.

Women are more susceptible to problems pertaining to hormones. No matter how little we eat or how healthy our diet is, if it doesn't balance out hormonal misfires then the efforts will be wasted for nothing. There are different signs of hormonal imbalances and often women fail to recognize that.

- Pre-menstrual syndrome
- Irritability and mood swings over little things
- Extra weight hanging around the waist/belly area
- Excessive cravings for sugar
- Easily stressed out
- Difficulty sleeping
- Overwhelming feeling

Women need to know that hormones control nearly all aspects of losing weight. They affect your appetite, food cravings, fat storage, food patterns and even gut bacteria. This means that when there's hormonal imbalance, nothing will work out well for you unless you address this problem first. Eliminating junk foods and exercising regularly have always been the experts' advice on losing weight, but with hormones getting all fired up, losing weight will be difficult.

So what is the solution to all these problems? Resetting your hormones is the answer.

### What is a hormone reset?

Every multi-cellular organism produces biochemicals that coordinate the way the body and the mind behave. These biochemicals are known as hormones. They play a crucial role in the human metabolism. They affect the way we energize ourselves, how we deal with stress, how we collect and store fat and maintain muscle. These hormones also play a role in our sexual functions. They help regulate sleep and they control our cravings. When there's a disruption of the digestive process, or when we eat something that irritates the digestive tract, the brain signals the stress hormone, Cortisol, to take charge. We then crave for comfort foods and sweets as the body's defense against stress. And if we fail to regulate the hormone levels, even with regular exercise, we will still accumulate unwanted fats.

The easiest and the most effective method to balance hormones is to reset them. This way, we ensure a healthy and stress-free life. The author of the popular book "The Supercharged Hormone Diet", Dr. Natasha Turner, studied ways on how we can enhance our lifestyle and facilitate weight loss naturally through lifestyle changes and proper diet.

## Chapter 2: Basics of Hormone Reset Diet

The fundamental principle of resetting your hormones is to ensure that your mind and body will be coordinated properly to allow healthy cell metabolism which will then result in weight loss and better health. The hormone reset diet dictates that in a period of 3 days, there will be specific changes to your dietary program. In order to reset your estrogen hormones, gut bacteria and liver, you need to eliminate alcohol and meat in your diet. Every 3 days specific foods that wreck your metabolism need to be changed into healthier alternatives to reset the imbalanced hormones in the body. Once the hormones are reset, your mind and body will begin to function in harmony and you'll start to truly feel good about yourself.

Only 3 days?

Well, the minimum time allowed for a metabolic hormone reset is three days. However, in some cases, a 5-days reset is allowed especially for people who shouldn't have immediate dietary changes. Still, 3 days is the ideal amount of time because it completes the cycle of resetting the 7 metabolic hormones in 21 days.

### How is Hormone Reset diet done?

The goal of the hormone reset diet is to synchronize the 7 hormones of metabolism: estrogen, insulin, leptin, Cortisol, thyroid hormones, serotonin, and testosterone. Here is an overview of the hormone reset (every 3 days).

- No meat and alcohol: Whether you are a meat eater or not, this reset is important to everyone. Eliminating alcohol and red meat in your diet resets your estrogen levels in the body.
- No sugar: After 3 days of not eating red meat and no alcohol, eliminate or in some cases, reduce sugar in your food intake to reset your insulin hormone and eradicate sugar cravings.
- Less Fruits: After another 3 days reset leptin hormone by not eating fruits for 3 days.
- No Caffeine: Caffeine increases Cortisol in the bloodstream so eliminating caffeine resets Cortisol levels and reduces your susceptibility to stress.
- No Grains: Not eating grains for 3 days resets your thyroid hormones which are essential in controlling and resetting leptin and insulin levels.
- No dairy products: Resets growth hormones and improves insulin
- No toxins: Detoxifying resets testosterone levels which aids in proper reset of insulin, thyroid hormones, estrogen and leptin.

After 21 days, you will notice that your metabolism transformed you from within and you will feel better than you have ever felt before. You will no longer have to constantly battle weight gain and stress and you will have better sleep. You'll also have better sex with your partner.

# Chapter 3: Metabolic hormones in the body and their role in Weight Loss

Hormones are the key to curbing metabolism. They can either reduce or increase cravings. If your aim is to get fit, hormones can reduce unwanted fats. If you want to lose some weight, controlling the flow and ebb of hormones inside your body reduces hunger. If you want to feel young and attractive, balanced hormone levels will help you achieve that. If you crave for a more rewarding sex with your partner, there is also a specific hormone to tap for that.

In this chapter, we will introduce you to the five most influential hormones in the body and the roles they play in the metabolic process. Dr. Lena Edwards of Balance Health and Wellness Center in Kentucky believes that people can control their hormones. She believes that we can make these important chemicals work in our advantage.

Let's take a look into the five most powerful hormones and how we can balance them out:

**Serotonin and Cortisol**

Serotonin is a healthy hormone in the body which regulates your appetite. It suppresses your hunger and calms you down when you are stressed out. There are some drugs used for weight loss that boost serotonin levels in the brain because of its ability to control appetite. On the other hand, Cortisol is the opposite. It is a hormone that makes us crave for junk foods when we are stressed out. It is the reason why we tend to over-eat and over-indulge in unhealthy foods when we are worked out. Cortisol makes us hungry for sugar and high-calorie foods.

How to balance it out?

Diet plays a crucial role in balancing out hormone levels in the body. Increasing intake of foods rich in folate such as spinach, asparagus, and lentils helps balance out serotonin and Cortisol levels. Depriving yourself of enough sleep also increases Cortisol levels so get enough rest to reduce it.

**Leptin**

Leptin is a hormone produced by fat cells. Just like Cortisol and serotonin, it plays an important role in appetite control when it is balanced out. Leptin resistance develops when there is an excessive fat in the body. This condition occurs when the brain becomes resistant to higher levels of leptin. The brain sends signals telling the body that it is starving forcing you to eat high-calorie foods. Metabolism slows down to compensate for the effect of the resistance.

How to balance it out?

To combat leptin resistance and make it work to your advantage, eat 1 cup of healthy vegetables before 10 am each day. This reduces the hunger and the cravings for high-calorie foods throughout the day. Furthermore, vegetables are rich in fiber, vitamins and antioxidants that can greatly decrease the swelling caused by leptin resistance which then speeds up metabolism, limit cravings and boost fat-burning.

**Irisin**

The hormone Irisin is produced by our muscle tissues and it is secreted through exercise resulting to effective burning of calories. This is a healthy hormone and recently, researchers discovered that Irisin has the ability to make white fat (unhealthy fat) behave like a brown fat. It also helps diminish insulin resistance.

How to balance it out?

Since Irisin is released by muscle tissues, exercise is the best way to balance it out. Increasing levels of Irisin helps in the production of more brown fat which then helps in burning calories. Regulating temperatures at home is also one good way to increase Irisin levels. Lower temperatures cause white fat behave like brown fat and dipping your feet into a basin full of ice water for a few minutes is found to be 15 times more effective in fat-burning than it did in a normal room temperature.

**Insulin**

Insulin is a healthy hormone and it is responsible for pulling out extra sugar in the bloodstream every time we eat foods rich in fat and sugar. Excessive level of insulin is dangerous and may lead to insulin resistance and diabetes. The former is a condition where the cells no longer respond to the hormone effectively.

How to balance it out?

Insulin levels can be controlled by cutting on the food intake that can instantly boost sugar levels in the body. Drinks that contain high sugar levels like sodas and artificial fruit juices need to be eliminated if not reduced. White foods like bread, rice and pasta can be changed into brown rice or whole grain versions. Foods that are naturally high in fiber slow down sugar absorption into the bloodstream thereby allowing insulin do its job more effectively. Another way to maintain healthy levels of insulin in the blood is to eat small portions of fiber-rich meals at frequent intervals.

# Chapter 4: How to Repair Hormones and Lose weight in the Process through Hormone Reset Diet

We already established that hormonal imbalance is often the root cause why most dietary programs don't work despite people's strict observance. We also said earlier that the only way to solve this issue is to balance out the metabolic hormones through the hormone reset diet. However, it is not enough that we know all these things. We have to know how to execute the hormone reset diet properly in order for all of these to work out. We need to know what specific foods to avoid and what are the better alternatives. We also need to be aware of our problem areas so we can easily target the fats and eliminate them through proper diet and exercise.

Solving hormonal imbalances takes more than just exercise and sleep. Diet and meal frequency is equally important. Some people choose to take supplements and artificial means but the natural way to do it is always better. Here are some effective tips on how to properly repair hormonal imbalance and lose weight.

### Detoxify

Just like how we start cleaning the house before we arrange and organize furniture, our body needs to be cleansed before we start resetting the hormones. We need to start the hormone reset by flushing out toxins from the body. There are certain food products that may irritate the digestive tract and this often causes hormonal imbalance. Consequently, food cravings are encouraged by the brain because the metabolism slows down as a result of the inflammation. As this happens regularly, your body starts to accumulate fat and store them away where you cannot eliminate them easily.

In order to detoxify your body, you need to eat foods that can prevent the onset of digestive tract inflammation. **Here are some foods to avoid**:

- Foods that cause allergic reaction like seafood, poultry, dairy products, and any food that may irritate your gums or throat or tongue even on a mild level
- Foods that have high levels of glycemic index as they contain high sugar and calories which increases cravings. These are white foods like pasta, noodles, processed food products, white bread, white rice and soda.

### Foods to eat:

- To keep hormones balanced, foods that contain low glycemic index are recommended.
- High-fiber foods such as artichokes, oatmeal, bananas, raisins, nuts and beans (whole grains) are very helpful in the prevention of digestive tract irritation.

- Water is a very important factor in detox. Always drink at least 8 cups of water on a daily basis to facilitate detox and boost metabolism.

## Target Problem Areas

We all have our own specific problem areas. Some people have difficulty eliminating belly fats; some don't feel comfortable about their buttocks, and others have fat deposits on the back. These problems areas need a lot of attention. Some people prefer to take on supplements that target these areas but there will always be a natural alternative.

## Belly fat

This is the most common problem that people face. We all want a flat belly with beautiful abs. We feel envious of the models on TV and in print because they can go around with skimpy clothing showing their flat stomach while we just sit in a corner hiding our belly fats.

Studies show that basil is a powerful natural product that can maintain healthy levels of Cortisol in the blood. Other foods that can be good alternatives to supplements are barley, citrus, spinach, beans and nuts.

## Buttocks

High levels of estrogen can cause your buttocks to blow out of proportion. Some people like to have big and shapely buttocks but if they get blown out of proportion, it is not healthy anymore. The best way to eliminate excess levels of estrogen is to eat vegetables like cabbage, cauliflower, and broccoli. These cruciferous vegetables are rich in phytochemicals that block estrogen. Polyphenols like sesame seeds, flax and chia, on the other hand, can get rid of excess estrogen in the bloodstream. To lower estrogen levels, you should eat red grapes and pomegranates.

## Back:

Apart from green-leafy vegetables and whole grains, foods that are high in linoleic acid such as beef and dairy products (cheese, yogurt and milk) can curb insulin levels at a minimum. It is not common to have fat on the torso and back but it happens and often it is a sign of high levels of insulin in the blood.

# Chapter 5: The Hormone Diet: Indepth Review

The claim behind the hormone diet is that most of the weight problems result from hormonal imbalance. Dr. Natasha Turner, the author of this said program, explains how the rise and fall of specific levels of hormone in the blood can cause accumulation and storage of excessive body fat. Not only does it cause weight gain, it also contributes to a lagging libido, health problems, sluggishness, sugar cravings and stress.

Dr. Turner encourages a 2-weeks detox and a lifestyle change to solve hormonal imbalance with a strict observation of Mediterranean-style diet with additional supplements. She believes that with this hormone diet plan, you can transform your health and energy levels and eliminate excess pounds in as early as one week.

**The Food Plan:**

The other term for the hormone diet is Glyci-Med which is a combination of foods with low GI (Glycemic Index) and the traditional Mediterranean diet. These foods do not cause rapid boost in sugar levels and so they don't increase the cravings. Here is a list of the foods that are recommended under the Glyci-Med diet:

- Vegetables
- Fruits that are low in sugar
- Flax seeds
- Chia seeds
- Lean protein like eggs and chicken breasts
- Fish
- Olive oil
- Nuts
- quinoa
- Unsaturated fats and oil like canola
- Whole grains like brown rice and buckwheat

Foods that are not recommended under the Glyci-Med diet:

- Alcohol
- Processed meat
- Caffeine
- Saturated fat
- Fried foods
- Foods high in GI like pasta and white bread
- Artificial sweeteners

- Peanuts
- Full fat dairy products

**Meal frequency**: 80 percent of the time, food choices are healthy and can be taken in every 3-4 hours. There is one or two "cheat meals" a week.

**Effort level**: Moderate to Difficult

It is never easy to drastically change your eating patterns and habits. The hormone diet restricts a lot of food products that a person can easily get attached to. You will be required to quit sugar, alcohol, caffeine, most oils, gluten and dairy for 2-3 weeks. This may cause problems to some people especially those who have a habit of taking these foods at frequent intervals on a daily basis. The body's pH balance also needs to be monitored. A series of tests also needs to be done to ensure safety and well-being of the practitioners especially on the first stage of the hormone diet. These tests include saliva, urine and blood tests to check hormone levels. Finally, the diet plan also recommends supplements like calcium, vitamin D3, magnesium, Omega 3 and multivitamins.

**Drawbacks:**

The hormone diet is a big adjustment for people who were used to eating prepared snacks and meals because the foods need to be prepared at home. Giving up alcohol and soda for example is also very difficult to do because not everyone likes to drink green tea.

**Shopping and cooking**: Organic foods are recommended. There will be a one week sample recipes provided and these are relatively simple. Options are also limited if you are not comfortable about the idea of foods on the diet plan and how they are supposed to be prepared.

**What sort of exercise is needed?**

Exercise activities like yoga, cardio, strength training, and interval training are advised for 30 minutes every day.

**Are dietary preferences and restrictions allowed?**

For those who are into gluten-free diet, the restriction is only up for 2 weeks. After 2 weeks, gluten is allowed in minimal amounts. Dr. Turner advises that it is good to avoid white rice and white bread and just eat their brown variants because they are healthier. And for those who are eating vegetables and lean protein, like the vegetarians and vegans, they have nothing to worry about because the diet is composed mainly of vegetables and some protein which works well for them. Any foods that may have a negative effect on the body after the detox phase need to be avoided.

**Is it cheap?**

Organic foods are more expensive than the foods that we normally buy in the supermarket. You also need to buy hormone tests which may not be covered by your insurance and some recommended supplements. So if you cannot afford additional expenses, hormone diet as recommended by Dr. Turner may not be a good option for you. The good news is, even without the tests, you can still finish the hormone reset diet plan in 2-3 weeks. The result will more likely be the same without the hormone tests because you can definitely feel the difference after the detox period.

**Is it effective in weight loss?**

Yes, it is effective in weight loss. The dietary plan consists of foods that are low in calories. Other positive effects of the Glyci-Med diet according to practitioner testimonies are:

- Better sleep patterns
- Healthy and glowing skin
- Healthier and vibrant hair
- Reduced stress
- Better sex with their partner
- And weight loss

However, some scientists believe that supplements are not really advisable if you are on organic diet. Organic diet is really healthy but there are still natural alternatives to good health and weight loss that are cheaper.

Glyci-Med diet or a low-carb diet in general offers rewarding results and benefits to most people. It helps improve health conditions like heart disease, hypertension and diabetes.

# Chapter 6: Sample Hormone Reset Diet Recipes

This eBook about hormone reset diet will not be complete without sample recipes. Beginners need to know how the food is prepared and which ingredients are best used for one particular meal. The recipes provided here are very easy to make and the ingredients can be found easily in the supermarkets.

### 1. Blueberry smoothie with goat yogurt

**Serving**: 1
Ingredients:
Frozen blueberries (½ cup)
Frozen banana (½ cup)
Plain goat yogurt (½ cup)
Chia seeds (1 tbsp)
Whey protein isolate (1 serving)
Water (1/2 cup)

### Directions:
Using a blender, mix the purée and all the ingredients together until the consistency is smooth.

### 2. Lettuce wraps and Crispy Chicken

**Serving:** 1
Ingredients:
4-5 ounces Chicken breast (boneless and skinless) – diced and cooked
Small Lettuce head
Cucumber (1/4 cup – diced)
Red bell pepper (1/4 cup- diced)
Unpeeled green apple (diced)
Low-fat Greek yogurt (1/4 cup)
Red onion (1 tbsp – finely chopped)
Virgin olive oil (2 tsp)
Pepper
Salt

### Directions:

1. Put the lettuce away and mix all the ingredients together in a medium-sized bowl.
2. Put the bowl in the chiller and leave it there for at least an hour.
3. After one hour, scoop the chicken mixture and carefully place inside each lettuce leaf.
4. Roll each leaf into cylinders.
5. Serve.

### 3. Tropical Smoothie

**Serving:** 1
Ingredients:
Water (2 cups)
Peeled Mango (cubed)
Banana (peeled)
Raw Baby Spinach (2-3 cups)

**Directions:**
Using a blender, combine all the ingredients together until consistency is smooth.

### 4. Pecan Candy
**Serving:** 1
Ingredients:
Pecans (2 cups)
Yacon syrup (2 tbsp)
Salt (1/2 tsp)
Olive oil (1 tbsp)

**Directions:**
1. Using a large bowl, mix all the ingredients together.
2. Set the oven at 350°F.
3. Put the mixture in a baking dish (9x13)
4. Bake the mixture for 15 minutes.
5. Let it cool for 5 min outside the oven.
6. Serve and enjoy.

### 5. Hearty Snack
**Serving:** 1
Ingredients:
Yellow pepper (chopped)
Carrots (Chopped into thin strips)
Celery stalks (Chopped into thin strips)

**Directions:**
1. Make sure that the carrots and the celery stalks are washed before cutting them into thin strips.
2. De-seed the yellow pepper before chopping it.
3. Place all the vegetables into a medium-sized bowl and chill for 30 minutes
4. Add salad seasoning or mayonnaise whichever you prefer.
5. Serve and enjoy.

## 6. Cashew-flavored Bread
**Serving**: 1 loaf
Ingredients:
Baking soda (1/3 tsp)
Honey (1 tsp)
Cashew butter (1 cup)
5 eggs
Apple Cider Vinegar (1 tbsp)
Salt (1/4 tsp)

### Directions:
1. Using a food processor, pulse the cashew butter and the eggs together until consistency is smooth.
2. Add in the apple cider vinegar, honey, baking soda and salt.
3. Pulse altogether.
4. Prepare a baking dish (8x4 in size) and pour the batter into it.
5. Set the oven at 350°F.
6. Bake the mixture for 45 minutes until it turns brownish.
7. Set it aside for 2 hours to cool down.
8. Serve and enjoy.

## 7. Energy-boosting baby spinach salad
**Serving**: 4
Ingredients:
Walnuts (1 cup)
Apple
Baby spinach (5 cups)
Balsamic vinegar (2 tbsp)
Olive oil (2 tbsp)
Currants (1/4 cup)

### Directions:
1. Wash all the ingredients together.
2. Cut the apple into 2-inch thin strips.
3. In a large bowl, mix the apple, spinach and the currants then set it aside.
4. Over medium heat, toast the walnuts for 10 min. until brown.
5. Add walnuts into the large bowl.
6. Drizzle the salad with olive oil and vinegar and toss it.
7. Serve it and enjoy.

## 8. Cauli salad with eggs
**Serving**: 2-3
Ingredients:
Celery stalks (chopped into dice)
Hard-boiled eggs (cut into cubes)
Cauliflower head (medium size)
Mayo (2 tbsp)

Onion (3-4 tbsp finely chopped)
Parsley (1 tbsp finely chopped)
Mustard (1 tbsp)
Salt (1/2 tsp)

**Directions:**
1. Wash all the vegetables first before cutting.
2. Cut small cauliflower florets about half an inch.
3. Blanch or steam the cauliflower until it is tender or until the aroma fills the kitchen
4. Transfer the cauliflower into a large bowl and set it aside to cool for 5 minutes.
5. Add in parsley, celery, onion and eggs.
6. Season it with salt and add mustard or salad dressing mayo if preferred.
7. Serve and enjoy.

## 9. Nutty Pumpkin Salad with zucchini
**Serving**: 4
Ingredients:
Yellow squash (thinly sliced)
Zucchini (thinly sliced)
Basil (2 tbsp – thin strips)
Olive oil (2 tbsp)
Almonds (1/4 cup – chopped)
Lemon juice (natural 1 tbsp)
Salt (1/4 tsp)

Directions:
1. Wash all the ingredients together before cutting into thin strips.
2. In a medium-sized bowl, mix all the ingredients: squash, olive oil, zucchini, salt, basil and lemon juice.
3. Set it aside for 20 min to 1 hr.
4. Add in the chopped almonds and toss it together.
5. Serve and enjoy.

## 10. Tomato-Carrot smoothie
**Serving**: 1
Ingredients:
Carrots (thinly sliced)
Tomato
Water (1/2 cup)
Whey protein isolate (1 serving)

**Directions**:
1. Wash carrots and tomatoes before cutting into thin strips.
2. Deseed tomatoes and cut into thin pieces
3. Blend together with the whey protein isolate
4. Add water and blend in together until smooth.

# Conclusion

Thank you again for downloading this book!

I hope this book was able to help you to learn all about your hormones and what you can do to lose weight effectively and efficiently. This book provides you with a clear understanding of all the hormones that play a major role in your body and day to day living.

There are a dozen of recipes and smoothies that are guaranteed to reset your hormone levels and detoxify your liver and body. Please follow these directions and you will see a MAJOR change in your health.

The next step is to take action. You can read all day, but if you want serious long lasting change, You have to take action and implement everything that you have learned in this book.

**Scroll Down To Check Out My other Books on Amazon!!**

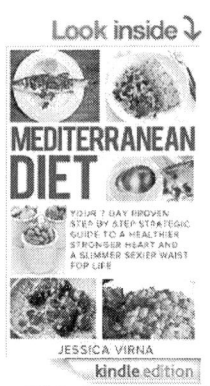

OR Enter This Link http://amzn.to/1dYnHnF

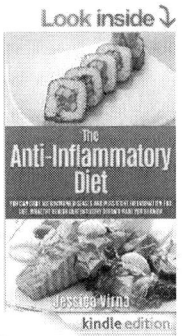

Anti Inflammatory Diet: What the Healthcare Industry Doesn't Want You to Know! Cure Autoimmune Diseases and Persistent Inflammation for Life Naturally!
**Enter This Link:** http://bit.ly/1K3bUln

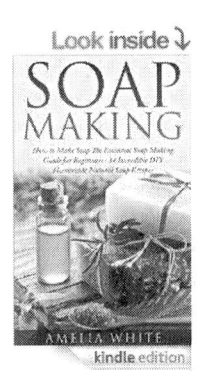

Soap Making: How to Make Soaps - The Essential Soap Making Guide for Beginners (34 Incredible DIY Homemade Natural Soap Recipes
**Enter This Link:** http://amzn.to/1IxIaer

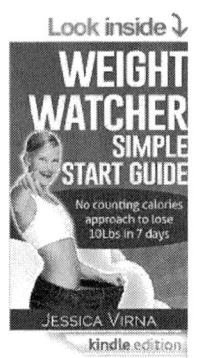

Weight Watchers: Easy START Guide and Cookbook - No Counting Calories Approach to Lose 10LBs in 7 Days. (Learn Exactly How I lost 140 pounds and Enjoyed Life)
**Enter This link: http://amzn.to/1dYoBR6**

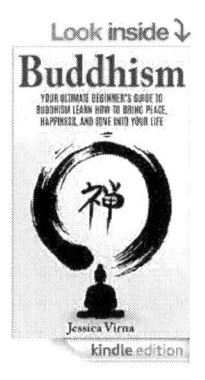

BUDDHISM: Your Ultimate Beginner's Guide to Bring Peace, Happiness, and Enlightenment Into Your Daily Life
**Enter This Link: http://amzn.to/1PfdmVd**

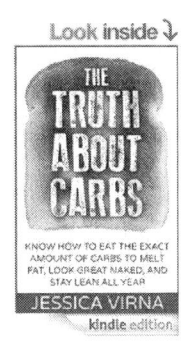

The Truth About Carbs: Know How to Eat The Exact Amount of Carbs to Melt Fat, Look Great Naked, and Stay Lean All Year
**Enter This Link: http://amzn.to/1QDIN8Z**

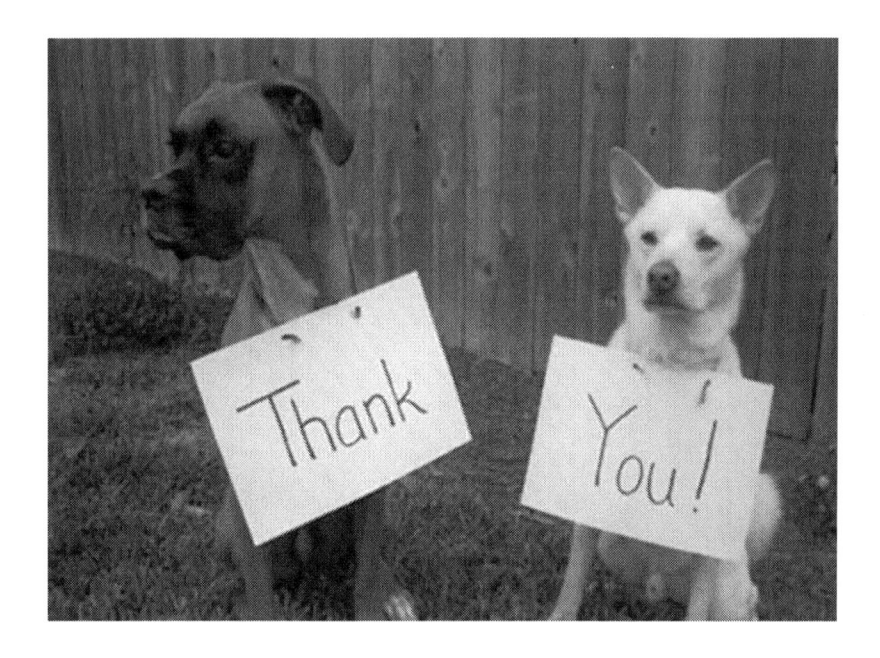

Finally, if you enjoyed this book, then I'd like to ask you for a favor, would you be kind enough to leave a review for this book on Amazon? It'd be greatly appreciated!

Click here to leave a review for this book on Amazon!

Thank you and good luck!

© **Copyright 2014 by Angel Publishing INC- All rights reserved.**

This document is geared towards providing exact and reliable information in regards to the topic and issue covered. The publication is sold with the idea that the publisher is not required to render accounting, officially permitted, or otherwise, qualified services. If advice is necessary, legal or professional, a practiced individual in the profession should be ordered.

- From a Declaration of Principles which was accepted and approved equally by a Committee of the American Bar Association and a Committee of Publishers and Associations.

In no way is it legal to reproduce, duplicate, or transmit any part of this document in either electronic means or in printed format. Recording of this publication is strictly prohibited and any storage of this document is not allowed unless with written permission from the publisher. All rights reserved.

The information provided herein is stated to be truthful and consistent, in that any liability, in terms of inattention or otherwise, by any usage or abuse of any policies, processes, or directions contained within is the solitary and utter responsibility of the recipient reader. Under no circumstances will any legal responsibility or blame be held against the publisher for any reparation, damages, or monetary loss due to the information herein, either directly or indirectly.

Respective authors own all copyrights not held by the publisher.

The information herein is offered for informational purposes solely, and is universal as so. The presentation of the information is without contract or any type of guarantee assurance.

The trademarks that are used are without any consent, and the publication of the trademark is without permission or backing by the trademark owner. All trademarks and brands within this book are for clarifying purposes only and are the owned by the owners themselves, not affiliated with this document.

Made in the USA
Monee, IL
14 May 2021